A CONVERSATION ABOUT ALZHEIMER'S

by

MICHELE L. TUCKER

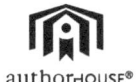

authorHOUSE®

AuthorHouse™
1663 Liberty Drive, Suite 200
Bloomington, IN 47403
www.authorhouse.com
Phone: 1-800-839-8640

First published by AuthorHouse 9/26/2008

ISBN: 978-1-4389-1558-6 (sc)

Printed in the United States of America
Bloomington, Indiana

This book is printed on acid-free paper.

DEDICATION

This book is dedicated to my mother who only loved one man; my father. Mom, may these words forever comfort you.

To those I love and those who love me…
When I am gone, release me, let me go.
I have so many things to see and do.
You mustn't tie yourself to me with tears.
Be happy that we had so many years.
I gave you my love. You can only guess,
How much you gave me in happiness.
I thank you for the love you have shown,
But now it's time I traveled alone.
So grieve a while if grieve you must,
Then let your grief be comforted by trust.
It's only for a while that we must part,
So bless the memories within your heart.
I won't be far away, for life goes on,
So if you need me, call, and I will come.
Though you can't see or touch me, I'll be near.
And if you listen within your heart, you'll hear
All of my love around you, soft and clear.
And then, when you must come this way alone,
I'll greet you with a smile and "Welcome Home".

-UNKNOWN

CONTENTS

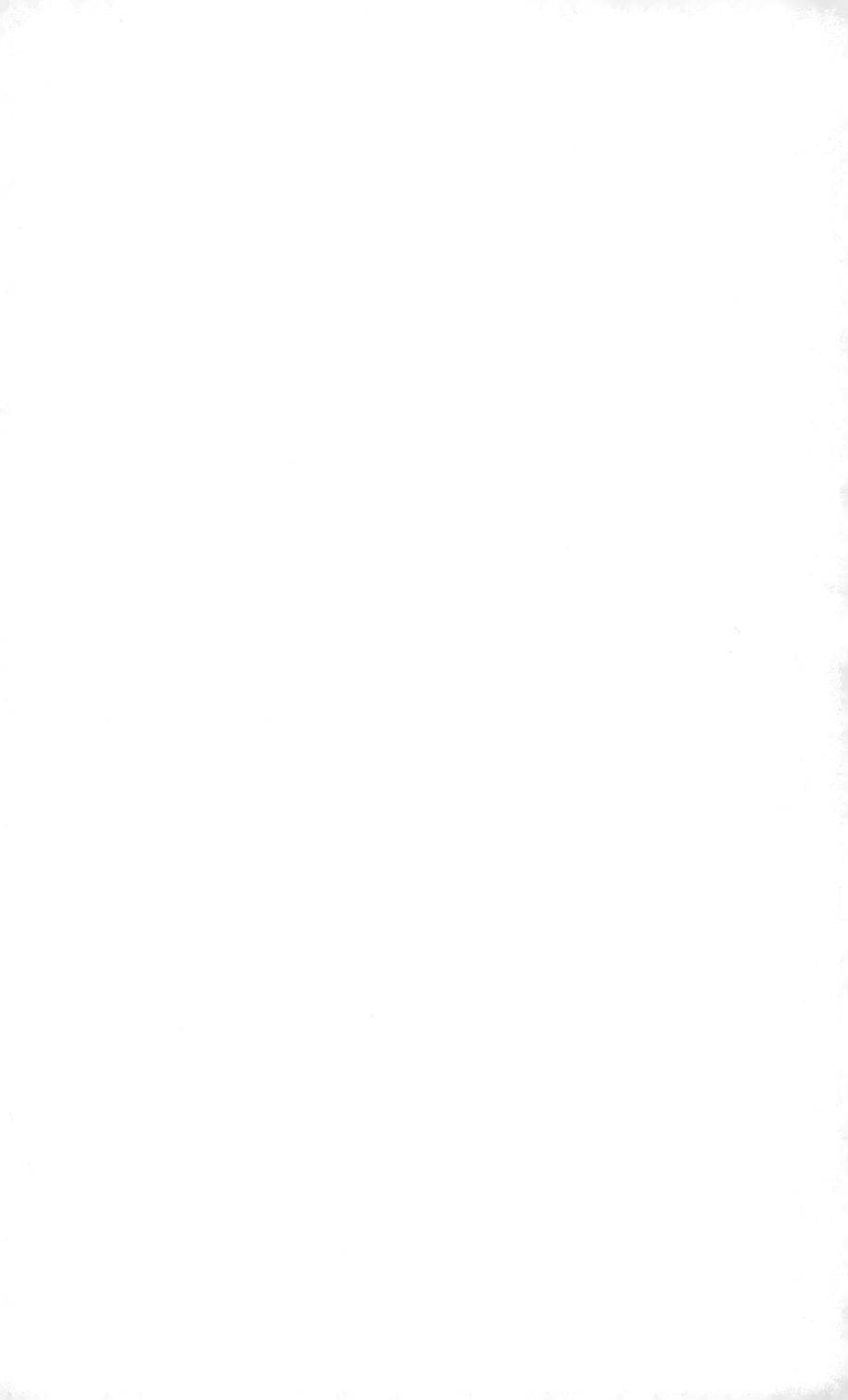

Hello

As with all polite conversation, let me begin by introducing myself. My name is Michele, I live in the state of Virginia and am my father's only daughter. This disease the medical community has dubbed *Alzheimer's* is not a dirty little secret anymore. Millions of people manage this new lifestyle every day. We each have our own set of coping skills, or so we think. No matter how little you know or how much formal training you may have, we are all flying by the seat of our pants on this one. Hopefully, what I have to offer, you will be able to use as a reference tool, a page you turn to when you need comfort, and an object you can throw when you are about to lose your mind.

It's a frightening journey we are embarking upon. Truly, each patient suffers in different ways; it's almost like a fingerprint. And that can be problematic in itself.

There is no blueprint, no template, no diagram to follow when taking care of an Alzheimer's patient – and let's face it, they aren't patients to us, they are our husbands, wives, grandmothers and grandfathers, aunts, uncles and siblings. There are so many unique stories and family situations out there. This is mine. I have tried to remain true, to the point of it being excruciatingly painful. But I feel I owe it to myself and to you as the reader. Life is not perfect nor are the diseases that we endure during our time here on earth. Whether your loved one has just been diagnosed or is in the mid to late stages of the disease, moments of clarity are held precious. My hope is that you find laughter and relief in the following pages; save the tears for another time.

My Experience

According to the American Heritage Dictionary, circa 1978, the word cruel is defined as *causing suffering, to inflict pain or suffering*. It is now 2008, and the definition of this word has not changed. This is the expression I use to describe Alzheimer's disease. When my father was formally diagnosed with Alzheimer's in September of 2001, I read every book, pamphlet, and newspaper article I could get my hands on. Educate, educate, educate… that's all I could think about. I told myself that once I knew the facts, I could get the right physicians, no matter the cost, to fix him. I just wanted to fix him!

The more I read, and the more doctor appointments I attended, the more I realized, there is nothing I can do to be prepared for what was about to happen. Of course there are handbooks for the caregiver on the bookstore shelves, autobiographies and the like. Each book, every website, offers phases of the disease, symptoms of the disease, how to relate to the patient in particular situations, but nothing exposed the real world experience.

Let's examine some of these unspoken realities.

A fact that seems to be locked away in some skeletal closet never to be discussed is the sad truth of losing friends during your time of need. When you hear of someone who has been diagnosed with cancer, the immediate response is, "I'm so sorry." You expect to see the person losing weight, losing their hair from chemotherapy with diminished strength. It's not the same with Alzheimer's.

This unfortunate experience of losing friends, and on occasion family members, doesn't happen to all. But this phenomenon does exist and must be brought to the surface so we can come to terms with its sadness and frustration. In most instances it can be chalked up to the simple fact of denial, but that's too easy.

The old saying that you find out who your true friends really are during a crisis is so accurate it stings. In a way, I don't think it's intentional. People are frightened of the unknown, they don't know how to act *or* react. What are you supposed to do when a person you've known for years, doesn't recall a special time you spent together, or doesn't remember your name? That's when the thought hits; I'm not going to put myself in that situation, that's how I will cope. Genius! Right? No.

I was witness to both the total denial of the obvious from family members and the noticeable absence of long time friends. My intention is not to name names nor to place blame on these individuals; rather to educate the sadness Alzheimer's can bring into your life, even from the unexpected.

I will say that the people I knew in my heart would be there for my mother and father were in fact nowhere to be found. I had co-workers that inquired more about my father than those closest to the family. I'm still left wondering why? I can only refer back to the definition of cruel.

As hard as it is for the friend or relative, consider how traumatic it must be for the victim of Alzheimer's. Can you for an instant, imagine yourself sitting in your favorite chair in the family room and suddenly not know where you are. You look to your wife or husband and say, "When are we going home?" What a terrifying moment that must be. This is a question my father often asked my mother during the early stages.

This is the reality of Alzheimer's; its unrelenting day-in and day-out effects robbing the victim every day of who they are. Quite frankly, the very fabric of who we are, *are* the memories of our childhood, teenage years, as young newlyweds and having children of our own.

The caregiver, they still have their faculties, what is to become of them? Truth be known, the victim here is actually the caregiver. The caregiver has all the memories both good and bad. They are now thrust into being chef, maid, financial analyst, landscaper, personal hygienist; when is it all going to stop? Unfortunately, I can't answer that question, the answer is too agonizing to let enter our minds, death.

There will always be people in our lives that come and go. If at all possible, reach out to those people that you hold dear to your heart and help them help you as the caregiver. Don't be ashamed by the actions of the Alzheimer's patient. We need to see them as their *new selves*; brain damaged and in need of love and attention.

Another aspect of the disease that is rarely spoken of is mood swings; let's ignore the outburst, it will go away. Typically, when speaking of mood swings we think of a child having a tantrum over a toy and just as soon as the toy is in their hands, life is good again. Mood swings for an Alzheimer's patient however, can be devastating to both the victim and caregiver.

A local nursing home was holding a free financial seminar to those people who have loved ones that are suffering from every type of dementia. My brother was kind enough to accompany my mother to the seminar. I was sitting at home that evening when the phone rang.

I hear this stern deep voice, "Michele!" I said, "Dad?" This voice sounded so angry. All of a sudden, my father replies, hysterically crying, "What is going on? Why is everyone leaving me? Are they taking me somewhere?" It was the sound of terrified desperation. All I could do was tell my father that everything was going to be ok and that I was on my way over to his house.

Luckily, I was able to reach my brother on his cell phone to tell him to turn around immediately and go back home. It's only about a 20-minute ride from my home to my parent's home; it was a ride of sheer panic. I convinced myself that everything was going to be fine once I arrived.

I opened the door and there my father stood, shaking and crying uncontrollably. He kept asking why my mother wasn't there. Over and over I explained that she would be arriving at any moment. I took him downstairs, sat him down in his favorite chair and gently covered him with a blanket. I sat next to him, speaking softly, trying to comfort his pain, but he could not stop crying. This is the strongest man I know. He is my father, perched on this pedestal that I created just for him when I was a little girl, and at that instant, *I was there to protect him*.

What was moments later, but seemed like a lifetime, my mother and brother arrive. As soon as they lay eyes on this man they've known as father and husband, tears stream from their eyes. My mind is swirling wondering how I'm going to handle this situation. I take a step back to allow my mother to hug my father, "Everything is going to be ok", she said. While watching my parent's embrace, I notice my brother standing off in the distance with his hand over his mouth, trying to stay strong, but crying just the same. But where were my tears? Am I so cold hearted that I have no tears to shed for this man I love so very much? There's got to be something wrong with me! Once everything was calm and the family was smiling again, I left. On the way home I continued to think, why didn't I cry?

When we are faced with tragedy, something mysterious takes over. We discover things about ourselves that we never knew could ever exist. I found strength that night, strength beyond my comprehension. Call it an adrenaline rush if you like, but it continues to flow through me to this very day.

Initially, I kept a diary of my thoughts. For one reason or another I stopped writing. I revisited my diary recently and felt it necessary to share myself with you.

July 22, 2002

I drove my parents to Mahwah (New Jersey) to see my grandmother, while she was staying with my Aunt. My grandma had tears in her eyes when she hugged my dad. I think it was very emotional for her now that dad has Alzheimer's. Since I'll probably be writing down the word often, maybe I should have an abbreviation – call it ALZ – like a stock symbol. It's almost been a year since my grandmother first called me about my dad. Obviously, several doctor appointments later, we now know it wasn't our imagination.

JULY 30, 2002

Talked to mom tonight. Dad had another – how should I say – outburst on mom today. He told her "it was about time they got divorced." Dad is truly coming out of his emotional shell with this disease. He no longer holds back what he wants to say, which I guess on one hand, is a good thing. It really makes me wonder though – these feelings he is expressing – are they his true feelings? Or is he angry over what he knows is going wrong in his head. It must be frightening for him - I only wish I could help somehow. Damn! I hate this disease! I wonder if someday Michael (my son) will be going through the same thing with me. With genetics and my head injury, I'm afraid the cards are stacked against me.

AUGUST 1, 2002

Mom and dad evidently had the biggest fight of their marriage last night. Mom's not ready to tell me what happened – too emotional.

AUGUST 8, 2002

Some bad news – found out what happened last week during mom and dad's fight. Evidently, dad has learned a new word; fuck. He not only said the "F" word, but said "F U" to mom – that has *never* happened. Dad was crying again. This is the 3rd time in one year that dad has broken down. I'm so sad for him. He's always been such a strong man. I still don't know how to help my mom.

AUGUST 13, 2002

Mom and dad bought a new car last night. Real nice. Had to help dad lift the hood so he could show me the engine. I never thought I would see the day that dad would have difficulty finding the lever for the hood. I'm starting to see a difference in him every time I visit. I hate ALZ, but hopefully since Charleton Heston made his speech regarding his situation, maybe it will bring some attention to this awful disease.

August 28, 2002

Had an out of control fit at work yesterday... slamming my office door and crying hysterically. What over? ALZ! I hate what it's doing to my father!

March 9, 2003 (last entry)

Well, it's taken me a while to get back to my diary. A lot has happened. My parents are returning from Florida one week from today. Can't wait to give my dad a huge hug. I just want him back home. They have been gone for 5 weeks now and evidently my dad's deteriorated considerably. I don't know what to expect upon their return.

As you can tell from just these few entries, my life was saturated with every emotion imaginable. It was a great time of confusion for me.

Ah, the Early Stages

The early stages can be quite a challenge. This is virgin territory. I will be honest with you – we didn't tell my father he had Alzheimer's until one year *after* his diagnosis. Was this cruel in itself? Not in our situation. If we told my father he had Alzheimer's, he would have been thrown into a violent storm of "when am I going to die?"

You see, in 1995 my father was diagnosed with Prostate Cancer. Naturally so, he was devastated; we all were. I was not about to sit around and have my father scared and lonely with his thoughts of dying every day. So I took action. I contacted the Discovery Channel who had recently at the time shown a program on a new prostate cancer procedure. Luckily, the physician who pioneered this procedure was in our backyard at Johns Hopkins in Baltimore, Maryland. I was able to play my role as *Miss Fix It,* Dr. Walsh saved my father's life and we lived happily ever after. Or so it seemed.

In the summer of 2001, my parents had taken a trip to visit my grandmother, my father's mother. The day after they returned home, my grandmother called me. I talk to my grandmother regularly, so the call was no cause for alarm, until she asked a particular question, "Michele, have you seen any changes in your father's behavior?"

They say there is such a thing as mother's intuition. Boy, whoever came up with that expression knew exactly what they were talking about. My grandmother went on to tell me about a particular incident that happened during my parent's visit. My father was pointing to something off in the distance; "Do you see that man over there?" he said. With my grandmother's keen 85-year-old eyes, there was no man to be seen.

During this visit, like so many others, they reminisced about the past, my dad's favorite thing to do. But my father's recollection wasn't as clear. Grandma said he was lying about things that had happened and *her* son does not lie. And not necessarily bold face lying, but exaggerating the facts.

What could be wrong? This is not like dad at all.

So I phoned my mother just as soon as I said my "I love you's" to grandma. I asked, "Mom, are you noticing anything different about dad?" "Yes", she replied. My world started to crumble. I didn't know whether to continue the conversation or act like it never happened and hang up. "Alzheimer's. Grandma said dad should be checked out for Alzheimer's", I said.

This was a very difficult time, how to proceed? My father is not the biggest fan of going to the doctor. Sure, he goes to the dentist and has his annual physical, but that's it. And he only does that because my mother will have it no other way. How on earth are we going to convince him to go to a neurologist? We decided to start out simple.

We made an appointment with his primary care physician. The doctor began the appointment by asking my dad a battery of what are supposed to be simple questions. "Please start at 100 and count backwards by 7", the doctor said. I'm thinking to myself, you've got to be kidding me! I'm 38 years old and putting way to much effort into answering the question myself. My father reached 93 and stopped.

After a few more questions, the doctor asked me to step into his office. Keep in mind I'm by myself with my dad, my mother was too upset to attend the appointment. We enter his office, he closes the door and says, "I'm sorry, you're father has Alzheimer's and there's nothing we can do". On the outside I accept what he's saying; on the inside I am screaming God no! The logical part of me is thinking, you haven't done a MRI yet, you haven't performed all the traditional scientific tests to *prove* it to me. You are wrong!

The doctor went on to recommend a neurologist for further testing. He followed up with my mother soon thereafter explaining there will be no further need to check my father's cholesterol and the like. Alzheimer's has made these important health statistics meaningless. Meanwhile, the drive back to the office from dropping my father at home was overwhelming. I cursed the doctor for being so forthcoming and bold in his diagnosis. I hated the doctor at that moment and thought he was a quack and needed a check-up himself.

Within the next week, the MRI results came back. Negative! The sense of relief was indescribable. I knew the doctor was too quick to judge. The thoughts kept lingering; there is something here, but what could it be?

Unlike so many other diseases, Alzheimer's can be a difficult diagnosis. It's a very tricky disease. It tries to fool you every chance it gets. Just when you think it's not Alzheimer's, the unmistakable signs come crashing back.

In the early stages, it's easy to talk yourself into *it's something else*. We have no family history of dementia, my father exercised daily both physically and mentally by taking walks and reading the newspaper, his cholesterol was pretty much nonexistent. The odds are in *our* favor.

At first, the symptoms are quite subtle, maybe a little memory mishap here and there. But let's explore what else this disease can disguise itself as; akin to a chameleon, it can change its colors quite rapidly.

There are so many boilerplate symptoms; it leaves you with many unanswered questions. What you read does not necessarily translate into what *you* are experiencing.

- Uncharacteristic outbursts of anger
- Vulgar language
- Becoming uncharacteristically quiet or more boisterous
- The television becomes a new companion
- Reading/comprehension difficulty
- Paranoia of family members stealing money
- Wanting a divorce
- Hallucinations of having a make-believe friend, seeing people or objects that are not real
- Crying for no apparent reason
- Loud noises suddenly causing agitation (i.e., volume from television or music)
- Difficulty dressing/undressing

If the above characteristics were rolled up into one big ball, you would have my father. From one day to another and at times, one moment to another, you would never know which behaviors would rear their ugly head.

Early on, my mother would not hear of "giving up". She would often force my father to write or sign his name in order to keep up this skill we take for granted. On this pink piece of paper he signed his name, but underneath wrote the following:

> I went down to the creek for a dive in the water,
> And all I came up with was mud in my face.
> I am old man without a penny to my name.
> Sometimes I think I'm going insane!
> I'm taking lessons to play the guitar,
> The only encouragement I get
> Is the man with the sitar!

It really makes you wonder what is going on inside his mind. Is he confused? Is he scared? Can he actually feel something in his head; a strange sensation? At the time it didn't make sense to me, but on several occasions my father confided in me that he knew *"something was wrong"*, as he pointed to his head. He just couldn't explain it in words. Although this poem is simple in nature, it gives you the impression that the author, my father, is a sad and lonely man.

In the initial part of the disease, my mom would put my father to bed and follow shortly thereafter. She would become so frustrated because his head would hit the pillow and would be out, snoring terribly. Quite often he would seem to awaken and reach his arm towards the ceiling as if grabbing something. Mom would ask him, "What is it?" "I'm trying to get these spider webs", he would say. Sometimes my father would see them so clearly that he would reach out and grab an imaginative handful and literally go to the restroom to put them in the sink. As this behavior continued, she soon learned that if she reached up with him and say, "I've got it", he would be satisfied and go back to sleep.

As it is with our normal personality traits, the Alzheimer's patient can suddenly alter with no rhyme or reason. What I refer to as the "silent treatment" may or may not affect your loved one, but during a particular phase, it appeared in my father. He was perfectly happy just sitting in his chair with nothing to say. Please don't think this is a *clinical* depression -my personal opinion is that it is one of those many characteristics that encompass Alzheimer's. It is also my belief that their minds just may need a resting period because of the chaos that is going on in the brain.

I beg of you as the reader, do not deny the signs. It is always better to be wrong then to allow the seriousness of the disease to go untreated.

Independence

It comes in many forms, this concept we call independence. Those of us who are blessed to live in this wonderful country, take this simple way of life for granted. Independence however, has another meaning all together when it comes to the debilitating effects of Alzheimer's.

It is routine for us to get up and drive to the store, drop off our children at school, or go to a sporting event. All of us are guilty at one time or another of complaining about rush hour traffic, honking at people to get them to move out of our way. Just going to the grocery store is considered a chore in our busy lives.

Try to envision one day your doctor, spouse or even child saying to you, "Hand over the keys, your driving privileges have been revoked". Not due to a faulty driving record, but because you have an awful disease and are now considered a danger on our roads, to yourself and others.

My parents drove everywhere. Neither would even consider flying, so all the years of vacations from coast to coast, were done on four wheels on the ground.

On one particular trip to escape the Virginia winter to Florida, my mom and her sister were in the car with my dad at the helm, on their way for a day of shopping and dining. My father turned onto a street going in the wrong direction. To be fair, all of us have made a wrong turn at one time or another, but this wasn't an isolated incident.

His driving habits started to change. My father began to drive faster, and even worse, he admitted to me, while alone in the car one day, to pulling over to figure out where he was. These were local roads he has traveled for over 40 years. Suddenly, these roads were unrecognizable.

My mom continued to express concern over his ability to drive safely. She had to tell him "left here", "right there"; he would become so angry, but knew deep inside he wouldn't know where to go without her directional assistance.

We discussed with the doctor our ever-growing concern regarding my father's decreasing ability to drive effectively. God bless him, the doctor had the daunting task of delivering the bad news to my father, no more driving. Wow! That went over like a lead balloon.

I can still hear my father yelling at the doctor, "Who are you? You can't take my license away! I have been driving for over 50 years and have never had an accident!" I knew then, this was going to be bumpy road; no pun intended.

Let me tell you a little driving story. I'm sitting at work one day when my mother calls. I hear, "Michele, your father has stolen the car!" Naturally, dreadful thoughts are running through my mind; *stolen* is such a violent word.

I asked her when this happened. "About an hour ago", she said. "Why on earth did you wait so long to call me and tell me?" I screamed. She thought he would have returned sooner.

So my mother called the local police department. They sent out two cruisers to the house to speak with her first. She explained to the officers that he had Alzheimer's and that his physician had revoked his driving privileges.

My father still had a valid driver's license in his wallet. Only the Division of Motor Vehicles and a court of law has the authority to revoke your driver's license. So in my dad's mind, he could still drive as long as he had that little piece of plastic in his pocket.

One of the officers sent the other out to look for him; he was traveling in a gold toned Volvo. The old adage comes to mind of trying to find a needle in a haystack. Not too long afterwards, here comes my father, cruising up the driveway with a "black and white" following closely behind; no flashing lights were used so not to confuse him.

He steps out of the car, my mother standing there with two police officers by her side. And my father's priceless reaction, "Hi, how are you doing? Nice to have a welcoming committee!" It was as if he didn't even realize these strangers were officers of the law. He even complimented them on how nice they were. You're probably wondering where my father went to. He drove to the mall and bought himself a frozen custard cone. He loved his ice cream!

The loss of independence was the single most difficult aspect of the early stages that we dealt with as a family. My father loved to drive. Seizing the keys to the car was traumatic to say the least. This compared to all else would cause fits of rage that I personally thought my father could never possess.

There are however, other modes of transportation such as a John Deere lawn mower that my father absolutely loved. He manicured his lawn and treated it as a trophy to be admired by all. As with the loss of his ability to safely drive a car, the tractor became the next target of repossession.

I recall one particular day going to my parent's house to assist with lawn care. While my mom did the trim with the push mower, I ran around on the green machine. My father paced on the brick walkway watching every turn I made. It was a moment of sickness in the pit of my stomach. Finally, I could no longer take it. I stopped the mower and let him ride it. I had finished the lawn so it allowed him to tool around. The prideful smile that came upon his face was priceless.

There are however, some positives of Alzheimer's in the early stages. I know what you're thinking. You've got to be kidding me; how can you make such a statement? I am now and will forever be daddy's little girl. My father and I have shared so much and I would never wish such a tragedy on anyone.

Some of you may not have had the best relationship with your parents, siblings, etc., who may now be in the unforgiving grasp of Alzheimer's. You have the power to completely change that connection into something wonderful and new. Given the opportunity to turn a negative into something worthwhile, isn't that the very definition of what life is? Don't be afraid of rejection take it on as a personal quest. It's an awful feeling to walk through life wondering if I only "shoulda, coulda, woulda".

This disease has altered my father's personality in so many ways – and yes, many are negative, but even in the darkest of times come the unexpected rays of light. He no longer hesitates to say what is on his mind. The disease it seems, has given him a new found freedom. We must not dwell upon the unpleasant, even though it seems our lives have been devoured by it.

Mid Stages

If you have not reached out for help by now, please do so. How could you possibly take care of someone else, if you're not taking care of yourself? My mother was extremely stubborn and would not reach out to her brothers or sisters. She solely relied upon me for venting her frustrations, her sadness and disappointment. It exhausted me. But I was there for her and my father throughout the duration of the disease. I kept telling myself that I never wanted for anything in my life because of my parents. It was time to return the favor.

Alzheimer's is a part of so many lives the options for assistance are endless. There are 24-hour numbers you can call to talk to someone about what you are going through. These people are very knowledgeable, most having experienced the disease first hand as a caregiver.

Of course, should you be fortunate enough to have family in close proximity, don't be shy to ask for some free time. It is very important that you escape the brutality of the disease. Put the guilt aside and think of yourself. It was simple with my father, all you had to do is take a walk or just sit and talk about the past. A family member would know what to discuss and therefore make the job of adult sitter easier. It's a fine line between asking for help and expecting it; be careful not to abuse those who do offer assistance. Remember, this disease takes a toll on everyone.

Another alternative would be to find an adult day care center. There are also organizations that you can hire part time in-home caregivers. With the in-home option however, there is no dispensing of medication. In-home care is mainly companionship for your loved one. They will also assist with light housekeeping and run errands for you such as grocery shopping. However, there will be a mileage surcharge for these services.

The most important aspect of what to do when asking for assistance is the comfort level of your loved one. Strangers can be frightening to an Alzheimer's patient. Thankfully, my father was a people person and not knowing someone had no effect on his behavior. Bringing in a stranger make take some time and patience for all involved.

I spoke earlier of what characteristics you may experience during the early stages of the disease. Let us examine the more difficult changes you may encounter during the mid-stages of Alzheimer's.

<u>Pacing.</u> Pacing can be a sign of agitation and or confusion. The person doesn't know what to do with him or herself. I say let them walk it off; it's two fold, they are receiving much needed exercise and as with a child, the pacing tires them. Be sure to inquire first why they are pacing; it just may be a matter of being hungry and they require a snack.

<u>Hiding Objects</u>. As with my father, many patients hide things. And not necessarily on purpose; they just like to find a new place these items. For instance, my father always did the dishes in my parent's household. He began to take the dirty dishes out of the washer and put them away; although in not so normal places. I think one of his favorite things to do was to hide the cars keys because he was no longer allowed to drive. Sometimes I wondered if he did so just to unnerve my mother – the mind is a wondrous thing to behold.

<u>Aggressiveness</u>. Not all, but some people with Alzheimer's can become quite aggressive even though they might have lived a life as a calm individual. I cannot emphasize

strongly enough that this is *brain damage*. The person cannot control what he or she has become. Certainly, there are drugs that can control this behavior and should indeed be researched and discussed with a physician. We had to put my father on an anti-psychotic medication to prevent his outbursts. He threatened on many occasions to strike my mother, but fortunately never acted out those threats. One evening though, my mother was in the kitchen bent over the dishwasher when he came in and kicked her right in the butt. We got a chuckle over it, but realized at the same time that his mind was deteriorating rapidly.

Argumentative. Whatever you do, do not argue with a person suffering Alzheimer's. You might as well be debating a brick wall. Their new sense of reality and history is just that; theirs. Go with the flow, and agree with whatever they are saying. If they are telling you a story about what happened 30 years ago, and it's a brand new version that you've never heard, listen and enjoy. Sometimes the new version is better than what really happened. One of my father's new stories was that he played with the New York Yankees even though the truth was that he only tried out with the Pittsburgh Pirates.

Repetition. This can be very aggravating to some. Listening to the same thing or being asked the same question over and over again. With my father, I would almost make a game of it. I would make up a new answer each time he would ask the same question; it kept it fresh for me and quite frankly, he could care less the answer I provided.

Sleep Habits. Sleep cycles can be thrown off completely during the mid-stages. You may begin to see your loved one sleep more often during the day and walking about at night. My mother didn't like the new sleeping habits, but soon came to realize it was time when she didn't have to be constantly looking over her shoulder to see what he was getting into. It was a time of peacefulness.

Support groups can also be of great help. Should you have difficulty finding one in your area, search your local church schedules. Many churches hold support groups and meet generally once or twice a month.

Now that I have mentioned support groups, it's not for everyone. Personally, I could never get my mother to attend. She felt embarrassed and frightened. She didn't want to sit there and listen to other people's stories of sadness while trying to cope with her own situation. I wholly disagreed with her on this point, but you can only take a horse to water; you can't make it drink.

During my research, I attended a support group held at a local church to find out firsthand what they had to offer. The stories shared were eerily familiar. The majority of these stories involved people having stroke-induced dementia and the patients were in their 80's and 90's. Since my father was in his 60's, it was difficult for me to relate. To be honest, sympathy was something I could not afford them. I could only wish my father would live to be 80, however I knew this to be impossible.

I also discovered in this particular group, many of the patients had issues with wandering. Not simply walking either, but utilizing for example, the public bus system to travel to other towns. The use of bells on door knobs or even an alarm system that would sound off when someone entered or exited a door is a useful tool to put the caregiver's mind at ease. Another *must* is to acquire a "return to home" bracelet. These identification bracelets are relatively inexpensive, but priceless for what it offers.

My mother and father lived in a tight knit community where everyone knew everyone else. At this point in the disease, this came in very handy. While my mother did not want others to know of his condition, I felt it very important to tell the world! I wrote the following letter and placed a copy in each mail box:

> Dear Neighbors:
> I feel the time has come to make you all aware of an important family situation in which we

now find ourselves. My husband, Tuck Masker, was diagnosed with Alzheimer's 2 years ago. This disease has unfortunately been progressing rapidly over the past couple of months. With that said, you may witness episodes in behavior that are not typical. For instance, you may find him on your property blowing off your driveway. He may also share information regarding his health condition. Due to the disease, some topics of discussion may come across as confused and illogical. I ask you to open your hearts and understand our daily struggle with this terrible disease. Should you have any concerns, please feel free to contact me at....

I cannot explain in words what a relief this was to my mother once it was made public. It was as if a big family secret had finally been told and we could all relax. This also helped tremendously with having more than one pair of eyes watching him should he feel the need to wonder off.

According to the Alzheimer's Organization, there are 7 distinct stages of the disease. And while it can be helpful, you must keep an open mind and realize that in *your* situation, this person may be showing signs from stages 1-4 full time, but on a part time basis demonstrating symptoms from stages 5 and 6. There is no structure to this disease and if you succumb to this fact, you will be in a better place for it.

My father loves country music with Hank Williams Sr., and Elvis being two of his favorite artists. There was a musical in the small town of Strasburg, Virginia playing. It was entitled "Hank Williams – Lost Highway", the life story of Hank Williams. When I saw the advertisement in a local paper, I immediately phoned my mother – wanting very badly to take my dad.

Keeping in mind that victims of Alzheimer's truly need familiarity in their surroundings, I thought my father would be fine since my mother, myself and especially my son accompanied him. It was this quaint little theatre – holding no more than 75 people per show. No matter what seat you had, it gave the feeling of being on stage. With the intimate setting, the actors could be heard whispering.

Upon arrival, my stomach was in knots. No, I wasn't embarrassed should my dad have an outburst; it was that feeling I always had – I just wanted him to be well again.

The first half of the show seemed to be enjoyable for all of us – even my father would scream, "Woo Hoo" over the excitement and stomp his feet to the beat. No sooner did he fall asleep with all that noise and began to snore. It cracked me up, but my mother kept poking at his leg to wake him so the snoring wouldn't offend those around us who also paid to hear Hank Williams sing.

It was intermission and time to take dad for a much needed restroom break. The line reminded me of something you would experience at Disney World in mid July. I was not shy when it came to his well being and comfort, so I walked up to the front of the line and simply explained to the person that my father had Alzheimer's and I would appreciate it if he could use the facilities next.

I guess I shouldn't have been surprised, but the look was written all over their faces and they welcomed my request with sympathetic eyes.

My mom gently guided my father into the bathroom and shut the door. I stepped outside, thanking these patrons on my way out, to get some fresh air. Suddenly, my mom comes screaming outside, "It's your father!" That 's all I needed to hear and went running to him. He recognized me right away saying, "Where am I Michele? What am I doing here?" I grabbed his hand and told him to follow me as I brought him back upstairs to our seats. I thought I was going to have a panic attack right then and there. All I could think of was I want to get him home; but the show wasn't over yet.

We changed seats with some very kind people, having moved dad to the end of the row should we need to depart abruptly.

The second half of the show began, but it wasn't the same. Instead of having a relaxed, snoring father, I suddenly had an anxiety ridden Alzheimer's patient. He was fidgeting and couldn't get comfortable with these strange surroundings. Ultimately, we left long before the show was over. His comfort was priority in our lives.

Sadly, we knew from the point forward, even if it was something my father would normally enjoy, we would have to be more careful in the choices we made when venturing out into the world that was no longer "normal" for him.

By this stage of the disease, sleeping quarters may be separate (as a necessity) for couples living this tragedy. Don't allow this separation to upset you; simply take it in stride. Focus on the big picture of keeping your sanity in check.

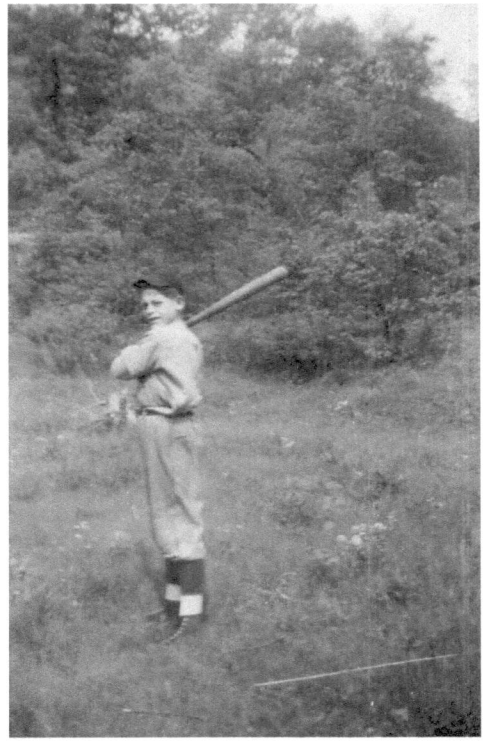

This picture is of my father as a youngster. He loved baseball and was so good that he was invited to the Pittsburgh Pirates to try out as a pitcher. Although he didn't make the team, it was a great moment in his life.

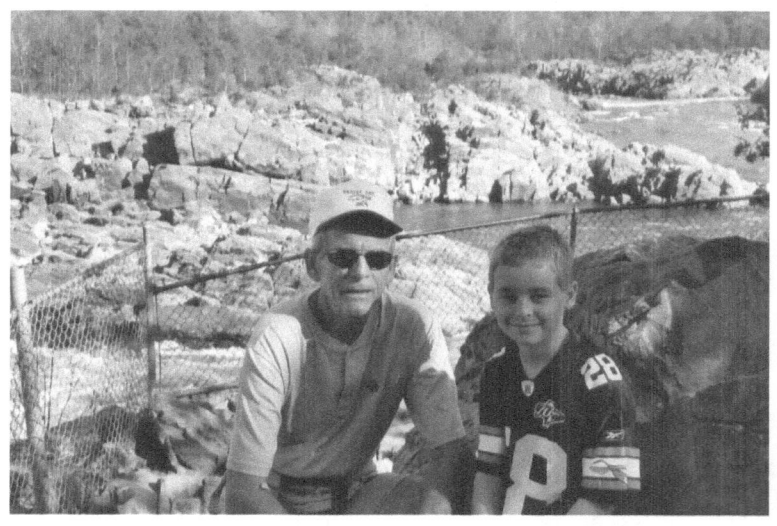

This is a picture of my father with my son Michael at Great Falls Park in Virginia. The love between them was indescribable.

alzheimer's ℚ association

Thank you for your patience.
The person with me is memory impaired
and may require a few extra moments.
Your understanding is appreciated.

National Capital Area Chapter   866 259 0042 **toll free**

This is a card you can request from your local Alzheimer's
chapter. It was a wonderful tool to have in your wallet when
out in public. Instead of having to explain an uncomfortable
situation to a stranger, you can just hand them the card.

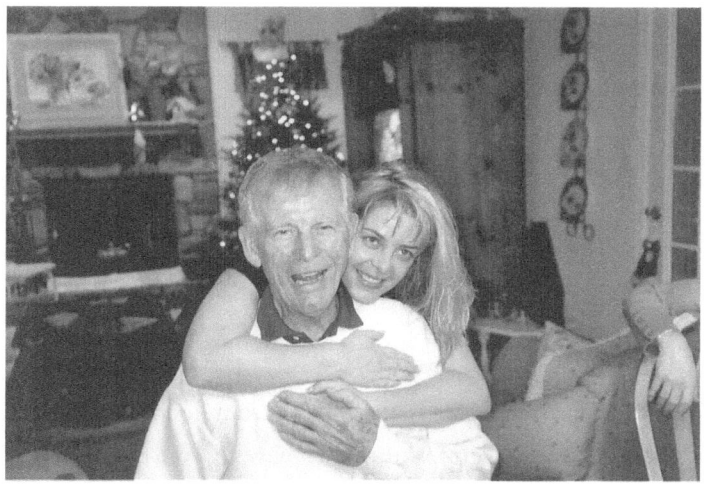

This picture was taken in 2004. It was the last Christmas I had with my father.

GUILTY, ANGRY OR BOTH?

Actually, this is a very difficult question to answer. You may have enraged moments, days or even weeks, but the feeling of guilt usually overrides. Are you allowed to feel angry? You bet! Do you know the reason why you are allowed to feel this way? You are angry not at the person, but at the disease Alzheimer's. Let's explore the different situations you might find yourself in and why, in effect, you are so angry. Your spouse may be the victim in this case, it's your golden years of retirement and you feel cheated out of the whole thing. You have worked, saved, raised your kids, and now this. I know you're out there screaming at the top of your lungs, "This is not fair!"

I know my mother felt this way; completely robbed of her future of playing tennis on beautiful summer days with my father. Future vacations were not going to be planned out and taken. Going to Florida to escape the winters, would no longer occur. No more leisurely visits to the Manassas Battlefield with the grandchildren to watch them run and jump on the cannons. It's over.

You may be an only child and your parent is the casualty of this horrific disease. You still have a full time job and a family to care for. Now you run over to the parent's house and fix breakfast; make sure they eat, take their medication and leave for work. Instead of taking a much needed "lunch hour" for your own sanity, you rush back over and bring lunch. Ah, the 5:00pm work bell just rang and you are doing what? That's right, driving back over to prepare dinner. This went on for months before the adult child finally hired some much needed daytime assistance.

I know of a family going through what I consider hell on earth. Picture this for a moment. You are a woman, whose husband dies of cancer, he is in his fifties. You are still working a full time job and your mother has Alzheimer's and your son (twenty-something) has been diagnosed with cancer. Can you imagine that tragedy?

We all have our situations, all of them different, but all of them the same. We are all in the worst of pain trying to cope the best way we can. When we feel depressed about our own situations, remember those who may have it much worse.

The word "guilt" sends shivers down your spine as a caregiver. Let's talk about what it really is to be a caregiver.

In our family's case, it was my mother taking care of a 175 pound child.

This person you've known as an adult may have been very independent or even somewhat dependent. No matter which scenario you experience, your wife, husband, mother, father, is now a new born person; reborn again in this adult body that can no longer learn. You may tell them once, twice or even three times to do something as simple as getting into a car. You may even go to the extreme of demonstrating how to get into that car. At that moment, not only can they not get into the car, but they are unable to learn how.

So here you are, trying to help your loved one, you're late for an appointment due to the day's confusion and it starts to boil. You can feel your face heating up – you can actually *feel* the color red. Boom! You lose your temper, cursing and saying things that normally may not surface. You scream, "Why did this happen to me? Why?" The new born adult just stands there and stares at you. Sometimes they understand and may start to cry; other times they just stare, seemingly having no idea of the current crisis.

In some situations, it is better to know that the person with Alzheimer's is oblivious to your outbursts. You don't want them upset; an upset Alzheimer's patient can be hell on earth.

You too?

As with cancer or diabetes, Alzheimer's has become the new disorder in which most everyone knows someone struggling.

It was a hot day in July, when I decided to visit an old family friend. Just a couple of weeks before, he had to put his wife in a nursing home. I had not seen this man in over 30 years, but now we have something in common; the sadness of watching a loved one endure the effects of this awful disease.

The reason for my visit was two-fold; to once again lay my eyes on this very gentle man and to listen to his painful story of acting as caregiver. The night prior, I had written down several questions in hopes that by only asking one would open the floodgates of communication. I also felt it intriguing to hear the view of the man who was struggling with the same caregiver demons.

I pulled into the driveway of this quaint brick rambler that was probably built in the 1960's; I could see him through the bay window getting out of his chair to greet me at the door. I could feel a rush of excitement as I made my way to him.

Before we sat down to talk, he took me on what I can only describe as an "Alzheimer's historical tour" through his home. He showed me where his wife's hospital bed was stationed in the middle of the family room. We walked down the hallway towards the bedrooms all the while pointing out pictures on the walls of his family; children and grandchildren.

To the left at the end of the hallway, we enter the bedroom they shared for so many years. Over to a dark wooden dresser, he slowly opened the top drawer, pulling out a picture of his wife from those "once upon a time" years. She's beautiful and lively in the picture. He shows it to me almost braggingly; I felt proud that he would share something so precious with me. I could actually feel the love this man has for his wife.

We made our way back to the living room decorated in perfect condition retro furniture and sat down. My first question was, "When was your wife formally diagnosed?" "September of 2002", he replied. As I had hoped, from that initial question, the story began to unravel.

While at the doctor's office for a routine visit, the doctor seemed a little more curious. She began to ask questions - rude questions it seemed. "Repeat after me. Say 'pen'. Say 'book'." The office fell quiet, because his wife lost the ability at that instant to repeat those simple words. Angry and humiliated, she quickly left the office.

This family is not so different from any other. They raised their children during the 60's and 70's; he worked as a construction worker outside the home, while she worked in the home taking care of the entire family.

I make you aware of this fact because suddenly, cooking meals, laundry, and all those typical generational "wifely duties" that she had performed for so many years, gradually became impossible tasks. The new "norm" was cleaning the floor from her accidents, feeding her, having to completely redress her because during visits to the bathroom she would *have* to remove every stitch of clothing. But with all these obstacles, she magically had the ability to put on her own shoes and tie them, "when she could find them", my friend says with a smile.

In 2003, the couple decided to drive to the west coast. They had talked about this trip over the years and knew with the nature of the disease, waiting was not an option.

She wanted to see the famous arch of St. Louis; her wish came true. They visited the Grand Canyon, Golden

Gate Bridge, and the great state of Texas. But all the while, she continued to ask, "When are we going home?"

He tried so hard to keep her home. She would sleep during the day and wander about the house at night. She would talk to her hallucinative friends and ask often about her parents.

She recognized her husband up until one month prior to her passing. She always greeted him with, "Am I glad to see you." But those words weren't spoken in the end. He had hoped that she still recognized her children, smiling at them, but seemingly unsure as to their identity.

What Should I Do When...

As it is with any situation, there will be several people offering advice on how to handle your new lifestyle. I thought it would be helpful to go directly to the source and ask people who have been living with Alzheimer's, what they would have to offer you as the reader. Interestingly, they often made comments about how they wished they had access to this type of information as it would have made their lives much easier.

- The number one piece of advice was to get the patient on one of the few available forms of Alzheimer's medications, such as Aricept®, at the earliest possible time. In most cases, it will stall for a while, the unstoppable.
- One vital aspect that should be addressed is your financial status. I suggest looking into a

Living Trust. It is an invaluable method to set up your finances. Do yourself a favor and research this sooner rather than later. My parents came very close to not being able to complete this transaction due to the fact that my father was losing the ability to sign his name. We learned of a Living Trust through a seminar that was held at a local Holiday Inn.

- Preparation is key when you have been dealt the Alzheimer's card. The reality of the disease dictates the necessity of making final plans for your loved one. Does the individual want a burial or cremation? Does he or she want their ashes spread in a particular location? Do you have a burial plot? At the end of this book, I provide a funeral checklist. This may sound morbid, but I can't express strongly enough how important this tool will be when the time arrives for its use.

- Laughter will more than likely be a strange concept to you as a caregiver. You will be so consumed by sadness and depression it will be a foreign occurrence. Let's face it, there's nothing funny about Alzheimer's, but there are funny moments. Allow yourself to laugh at times and don't feel guilty for it. Remember, laughter is allowed.

- Don't make the mistake of ignoring signals of memory loss! Take charge and schedule an appointment with your doctor immediately. In our situation we had no family history of dementia or specifically Alzheimer's. My father has now begun the tradition of this disease in our family. If you see a difference in a friend, a family member, etc., for God's sake speak up.

  We don't always see things clearly when we're so close to the person; such was the case with my mother. Of course she noticed little things, but it took a comment from my Grandmother to bring it to the forefront.

- In the majority of cases, Alzheimer's disease affects the elderly and more than likely, these patients will have grandchildren in their lives. When a person changes so dramatically, as with the effects of Alzheimer's, it can be quite frightening to a child; they don't always have the ability to understand. With this in mind, I asked my son (11 years of age at the time), what advice he would give other children who have a grandparent suffering this disease. And I quote, "To never give up on him and always love him. Don't think he's weird because he has a disability – help him and walk him through it. If you love him and hang out with him, he will never forget you – and that's what is important."

LATE STAGE...

According to the Alzheimer's Organization, it may take your loved one up to 20 years to reach this point in the disease. However, I sincerely hope this is not your situation. My father reached the late stage by year 4. And while this is very sad, there is nothing we or the medical community can do about Alzheimer's, so personally I would rather see the disease progress fast for the sake of all concerned.

Notwithstanding the effects the other stages have had on you and your family, the late stages can only be described as horrific. You are now completely helpless. The disease has taken its toll on your emotional as well as physical well being. You are experiencing these issues on a constant basis now:

Bathroom. The days of using the bathroom facilities independently are over. The use of an undergarment is mandatory and my sincere hope is that your loved one has accepted this demeaning new way of life. It is embarrassing and frustrating for an adult to have to in effect wear a diaper. But by the same token, by this stage, your victim is not even aware of having to use this garment. This protection is not always fail-safe. My father would often take off the garment and leave it lying in the floor not knowing what he had done.

Sleeping Habits. Speaking from experience, your loved one is most likely sleeping more than he or she is awake. I know my father drooled quite often while sleeping and had to be watched due to the risk of slumping dangerously or falling out of the chair. He had the ability to sleep the majority of the day and still have no problems falling asleep at night. The one big difference from mid-stage sleep disturbances was the fact that my father would awaken up to six times per night. Sometimes, he would say he needed to use the restroom; other times he wanted to be out of bed "just because". This was exhausting on my mother. Each time he would awake, my mother would be awake.

Eating Habits. Although my father's eating habits did not change (he would eat anything put in front of him), his ability to feed himself was dissipating. He no longer knew how to eat corn-on-the cob. He would pick at it with a fork. My mother would have to literally demonstrate how to eat it; sometimes it worked, sometimes it didn't. It became a necessity to cut up his food; using a knife was impossible at this stage. Also at this stage, choking on food becomes a real-life hazard. Did you know that many people with Alzheimer's choke to death? Their brains literally forget how to swallow. This is one of the leading causes of death for many victims. The very thought is terrifying.

We miss the early stages now. If your loved one is in the early stages, as strange as this may sound, take advantage of every moment. Make those reservations and take that trip that you always wanted to, visit every friend that you have missed, and plan the family gathering that you have been postponing for too long.

Nursing Home or Assisted Living or Home Care

This is the most difficult decision you will ever make in your lifetime. It's not only harsh on your soul, financially it can be life draining.

I had found this wonderful adult day care center close to my parent's home. It was becoming increasingly difficult for my mother to leave my father home alone and unattended – just as you would never leave an infant. She was able to run quickly to the grocery store, but never go out for more than 30-60 minutes.

It seemed that as soon as she would leave, my father would get into something. Granted, he would never turn on the stove or do something to endanger himself, rather, he would raid the sweets. The aluminum foil was found removed from the cake, but instead of cutting a piece, my father would just grab a handful and eat it. Times like these would bring a smile to my mother's face.

In 2004, we tried to have my father attend an adult day care center; just hoping and praying for 2 days a week. Although in the mid-stages of the disease, he still knew enough to know that he did not like it. At 68, he would say to me, "Those people there are so old." Unfortunately, my father's highly negative reaction towards the center won out and he remained home with my mother.

As with Alzheimer's, time went on and my father deteriorated. It was 2005 and we decided to give the adult day center one more attempt for my mother's self-preservation. Our patience paid off and my father absolutely loved the center. He would ask my mom, "Am I going to work today?" That's how he would to refer to the center. I guess it was his way of feeling he was contributing to the household, by *going to work* in his mind that was now engulfed in plaque and tangles.

I wanted my son to see his Grandpa and experience what the day care center offered to seniors, since he was so accustomed to child care centers. On this particular day, it was a surprise visit, like on so many other occasions.

My father's eyes glowed at the sight of my son. We sat in a quiet corner so we could talk without interrupting the other activities. Suddenly, an employee announced it was time to stand and say the Pledge of Allegiance.

I quickly grabbed my dad's arm and helped him out of his chair. "Come on Dad, it's time to say the Pledge of Allegiance", I said.

I pointed out the flag hanging over the fireplace; he turned and put his hand over his heart. And to my shock and awe, he said that Pledge, word for word, without hesitation. It brought prideful tears to my eyes. Afterwards, his diseased brain reappeared, struggling to get a sentence out clearly.

Not too long after, maybe a couple of months, we began receiving little comments here and there from the day care center providers. It boiled down to the fact that his condition was becoming too much for them to handle. Increasingly, my father needed special care of which the facility did not offer.

I remember his last day at the center. The faculty gave my father a going away party; nothing fancy, but you would think that he was the most special person in the world that day. He was able to remember enough of the party to express his joy to my mother. "They all clapped for me!", he told her.

During his last months of attending the day care center, I held more frequent discussions with my mother about next steps. I knew the day would come when she could no longer care for him, and I did not want to see that day unprepared.

We began the search for a nursing home; one that was within close proximity, reasonably cost effective with an impeccable reputation. You might as well be looking for the Holy Grail, this venture seemed virtually impossible. Needless to say, living in the Northern Virginia area, one of the most expensive areas in the U.S., the challenge was difficult.

The Internet can be a wonderful tool in searching for a home. The phone calls, the site visits, the referral checks must be done the old fashioned way and is tedious to say the least. It is however, a necessary evil that will pay off in the long run.

A checklist of what your requirements are is the best way to begin the process. In order to accomplish this task, you must be truthful or failure of the worst kind will surely follow. Ask yourself:

- What condition and or stage is your loved one in?
- What abilities do they still possess? (i.e., can they feed themselves, can they walk unassisted?)
- What is your comfort zone financially?
- How far are you willing to travel to visit?
- How often will you visit? (Be honest here)
- Private or semi-private room?

My father is now skimming the late stages of the disease. What does this mean for him and my mother? My father can no longer brush his teeth, bathe, shave, or dress himself. His eyes are in a constant state of being glazed over and his smile is no longer broad. His speech has deteriorated so badly, that it is a struggle to understand what he is trying to communicate. He is incontinent and has to rely on wearing Depends® undergarments 24 hours a day.

After much painful deliberation, we decided to put my father in an assisted living environment. Each family will handle this process differently. Once we found our first choice facility, my mother took my father for a site visit. It was important for us to see my father's reaction; after all, it was he who would be residing there.

The facility was beautiful. It was a private home, situated on 3 acres with a cozy gazebo near the front entrance. A small private room was waiting just for him – only thing missing was a few homey touches and his favorite chair. The property and residents enjoyed multiple daily visits from the local herd of deer.

It was Saturday, October 1st, 2005 and we were driving down Harry Byrd Highway, bags packed. I knew this was going to be one of the most emotional days of my life. My stomach was in my throat and I feared that one of my infamous panic attacks was brewing.

We made it a family event. My mother of course, accompanied by my brother, sister-in-law and the three grandchildren, myself and husband were all in attendance. We unpacked the vehicles and quickly furnished his room while taking turns keeping my father distracted. We hung family pictures, pictures of my father's dog whom he loved so much, and placed his chair next to the window.

Once finished, we had the unveiling and escorted my father to his new room. He seemed happy and content. We sat him in his chair in hopes of providing extra comfort to his frail mental state. I sat on the floor next to my father, keeping my hand on his knee. My niece sat on the bed with her mother having a difficult time holding back the tears that were streaming down her face.

Out of the blue from my father comes the following statement: "I guess it's time to move on and start a new life. I like it here". You can have pushed me over with a feather! Where did that come from? Why did he say it? Is there still enough comprehension in his brain to process something so complex yet that is so simplistic for you and me?

My brother was standing at my father's side, rubbing his shoulder; I could feel something was wrong. Suddenly, my brother leans over to hug my dad; his body shaking with each tear that fell. I could see my father's face through an opening. I was so fearful that my dad would suddenly realize what was going on and break down himself.

The look on my father's face surprised and saddened me. It was simply expressionless. His poor damaged brain could not comprehend this day that was eating away at the insides of his family. My brother exited the room and I was left there to watch my other family members cry while trying all the while to make my dad laugh.

It happened again. Another tragic family circumstance and I am not crying. Why am I reacting this way? I was solely concentrating on my father's well being and those family members surrounding me that I wouldn't give in to it. And even if I did, I don't think the tears would have shown.

The ride home was a quiet one. It was almost funeral-like. No one needed nor wanted to speak of what had just happened. Everyone knew the end was coming and no one had control over that fact.

According to the Webster's dictionary, circa 1988, the definition of the word heartache is a*nguish of mind; sorrow*. This is now my state of being. I struggle daily with the sorrow of what Alzheimer's has brought into my life.

IN THE END...

It was the evening of October 21, 2005 and I'm on my way to Wegmans® – a local up-scale warehouse grocery store. You see, I'm going to visit my dad tomorrow along with my mother and son, and I wanted to buy him something special. I found these magnificent muffins: one pumpkin chocolate chip, the other blueberry.

It is 8:45am, Saturday, October 22nd, my brother's phone is ringing. He answers and can barely make out the words my mom is saying, "He's not breathing." He asked her to repeat the words to make sure he heard correctly. My mom is crying in a way that my brother can only describe as "dry hysteria". My brother's first thoughts were that he needed additional information so he ran to my mom's house, enters through the garage and my mom greets him with, "They called and said he's not breathing."

My brother, called the assisted living home to speak with the owner. She explained how at the predawn check, my father was sleeping fine and snoring as usual, as well as at the pre-breakfast check. Upon returning to get my father out of bed to prepare him for his morning meal, they found him not breathing, but also not struggling to breathe. She went on to tell him that the paramedics were trying to clear is air way. He said "Okay, as soon as it is clear, call me."

It's now 9:06am, Saturday, October 22, 2005 and my phone is ringing. I thought it was my grandmother calling who had left a message the prior evening. She always calls me between 9-9:30am Saturday mornings. It was my mother calling. "Michele?" "Hey Ma", I replied. Thinking that she was calling to discuss our visit, I was about to tell her to call me back later because I was asleep. I could hear her crying when suddenly, "Hello?" It's my brother's unmistakable deep voice. I could feel a rush go through my body. I just knew something was wrong.

I literally fell out of bed and started crawling on my hands and knees across the floor awaiting my brother's news. "Dad is having trouble breathing, they are trying to open his airway now". For a moment, I thought to myself, "No big deal. The paramedics are there and he will be fine." I'm listening to my brother intently, but at the same time not letting the information sink in for fear of losing my mind. Then he spoke these words, "Dad hasn't been breathing for about 30 minutes now". I knew then, there was nothing anyone could do. We were still awaiting a phone call from the assisted living home to confirm his condition; dead or alive. I told my brother to hang up and call me as soon as they heard any news. I paced around the house, not really knowing what to do with myself; thinking that maybe this phone call never happened and it was all a horrible dream.

While I was awaiting an update, my brother was taking on the role of insulator rather than fact gatherer with my mom. The phone rang once and my brother abruptly picked it up and took staircase after staircase until he reached the basement of the house. He knew if it was bad news, there were many questions he had and did not want to ask them in front of my distraught mother.

The owner went on to tell my brother, "He didn't make it, I'm so sorry". He asked the what, why, when and how, but it was too soon to even know the answers, that would come later from the medical examiner. It was now time to leave the basement and take what seemed to be the walk of eternity to tell my mom the news. He walked up to her, hugged her, she slumped at the tragic news. "He was all alone", that's all my mom said.

Within 10 minutes the phone rang again. I knew it was my brother, but did not want to hear what he had to say, so I had my husband answer the phone. As they spoke, my husband kept repeating, "Ok, ok." Although it was a brief conversation, it seemed like time would never end. My husband disconnected the phone, looked at me and said, "I'm sorry, your dad is dead".

All the while, I didn't even remember the fact that my mom, in accordance with my father's wishes, had a DNR order on him. That's right, Do No Resuscitate. But they tried; they literally tried to save my father's life even though this order was in place. To this day, I'm really not sure as to why the owner of the assisted living home along with the paramedics, went to all that trouble to save his life. I can only assume it's a natural reaction as humans, not wanting others to die no matter what the paperwork may state. My father was in the assisted living home 3 weeks to the day when he passed. He died of a massive heart attack. And although it was the worst moment of my life, I will forever be thankful for these things: he passed in his sleep, he still remembered me, and he never reached the point of being in a vegetative state, which happens to so many others.

Sometimes I feel as though my father died on purpose to save his family the agony of watching his absolute deterioration. He would not allow himself to arrive at the point of having no family recognition or worse, the state of no longer being a person, just a body lying in bed waiting for the Lord to come and take him home. This passage has been an incredible one for me and my family. We've learned a great deal of how sophisticated the brain actually is. We've also learned how the brain can rip away your very existence. But mostly, we learned patience. With Alzheimer's, it tests your ability to be more understanding, kinder and gentler as a person.

The day after we buried my father, I took my mother and son back to the cemetery. My mom did not get close enough to the casket to look at all the flowers and notes that had been sent. The obvious stress she was experiencing at the funeral was too much for her to bear. I started to point out the different arrangements and reading the notes that accompanied each. She began to make comments when suddenly I asked her to stop speaking and pointed off in the distance. It was a deer.

As beautiful as this deer was, something was strange and out of place. The deer was actually walking *towards* us. I don't know what your history has been, but I have never seen a wild deer purposefully approach humans. Then it came to me.

I said out loud for all to hear, "Dad, is that you?" This animal came within ten feet of us and stopped. It stopped and stared as if it wanted to say something. To this day, I believe it was my father standing there to let us know that he was in a happier place; suffering no more.

I was told later that a deer represents unconditional love. That's what I will always have for my father; that great love if you are fortunate enough in life.

I will leave you with my eulogy. My thoughts and prayers are with each and every one of you out there that are currently or have in the past, suffered this awful fait of watching a loved one live with the cruel effects of Alzheimer's.

EULOGY

From a Daughter to her Father

October 27, 2005

It was 9:06am Saturday, October 22nd when I received the worst call of my life.

The death of a loved one is the ultimate in suffering. Truly, there are no words to describe how you feel. The afternoon of my father's passing, I had a moment to rest – and as I lay there, I could feel my chest tightening. But this feeling was different – it wasn't a panic attack, it was pure heartache. My heart simply aches over the loss of my father.

For all of us here, we have shed a tear, or several, but once those tears dry, we reflect on our memories of my father. When these memories come flooding in, it brings a smile to our face. May those memories stay with you forever and comfort you through this most difficult of times.

I want to share a secret with you that I have been keeping for over four years now. When I first learned of my father's diagnosis of Alzheimer's, my very first thoughts were purely selfish. Instead of thinking, "how am I going to make him well again?", my thought was this: Who is going to protect me now? But in the end, it was me who was protecting him.

My grandmother could not be here today. It is unnatural to bury your own children. My father is the second of her 2 sons to pass before her. As we all gather in this room, my father is with his mother at this moment watching over her and comforting her – that's just the type of person he was. So instead of speaking on her behalf, I would like to read to you a card she sent to my dad while he was at the assisted living home.

"Dear Tuck, It's a dreary cold day here today. A good day to use the rocking chair in front of the fireplace and think back of what used to be. I do this many times. I also like walking in a light rain and think about our family and the good times we had – sad times also. I dream a lot about the rain with you and Alfred protecting me finding shelter for me. You know Son, I'm a very fortunate mother in having such a lovely family, so kind, loving and considerate. Thank you Dear Heart. I love you. Mother"

To my niece Kerry. Papa literally stood right outside the door when you were being born. The moment he laid eyes on you, he loved you more than you know.

To my nephew 'lil Tuck. You have been blessed with Papa's baseball abilities. He will be there at every game for the rest of your life and I know you will make him proud.

To my son Michael. You had a very special relationship with Grandpa. I want to thank you for your love, patience and understanding throughout his illness.

To my Mom. Thank you for taking such wonderful care of Dad. I hope it brings you comfort knowing how much he appreciated everything you did and how much he loved you.

To my brother Tuck. You are our father's namesake. He was so proud of you. He loved the child you once were, but equally as important, he respected the man you turned out to be.

Finally, to my Dad. I have no regrets. I loved you the best I knew how and you gave that love back to me tenfold. I am now and will forever be daddy's little girl. I will miss you.... and I love you.

Funeral Checklist

The following funeral checklist was created by a dear friend and former superior of mine. He was the unfortunate soul to see his aunt and uncle pass within months of one another. He was the executor of their estate. Though sad and morbid to think about, death is a part of life. We all should be prepared for the inevitable.

Description	Approximate Cost
Mortuary/Funeral Home Selection • Referral from Minister • Referral from family friends	No Cost
Funeral home will work with hospital to remove remains and perform necessary preparations • Further transportation arranged by Director	$3,000-$5,000
Location of Service • At church where priest resides • At chapel on-site funeral home	Included Above
Burial Plot • Select site: single or multiple plots • Particular location guidelines: position relative to other family members • Obtain deed and receipt	$500-$2,000
Casket • Funeral home will have selection on-site • Caskets can be ordered with one-day turnaround out of catalog at funeral home	$2,500 - $10,000
Vault • Steel: galvanized or painted • Concrete • Special metals and copper	$1,000-$2,500 $1,400-$4,000 $6,000 +

Flowers • Augment those sent by friends and family • Central arrangement for top of casket	$300-$800
Obituary Notice • Drafted by family • Submitted through Funeral Director • All papers that matter (usually 2-3 papers)	$20-$200 Per listing
Guest Register/cards/flowers • Provided by Funeral Home • Collect all cards with flowers: instruct funeral home to write description of each arrangement on back of sympathy card	No Cost
Seating at Service • Family to sit in separate area • Pallbearers (active) sit in separate area	No Cost
Seating at Cemetery • Family in front • Pallbearers stand with other guests	No Cost
Bagpiper (optional at grave side)	$100
Music for service • Funeral home can assist with music choices	$100

ESTATE MATTERS

Death certificate
• Prepared by funeral home: need 10 copies

Liabilities
• Hospitalization and incidentals
• Credit cards
• Mortgage
• Other loans
• General unsecured debt (e.g. phone bill, utilities, etc.)

Assets
• Insurance proceeds
• Life (policy, employment, other)
• Health insurance reimbursements due

Checking, savings 401(k)
• Identify via executor letter
• Consolidate to master account for liabilities

Property
• House
• Auto
• Brokerage Accounts

Probate
• State laws, safe harbor
• Executor's note
• File and wait

About the Author

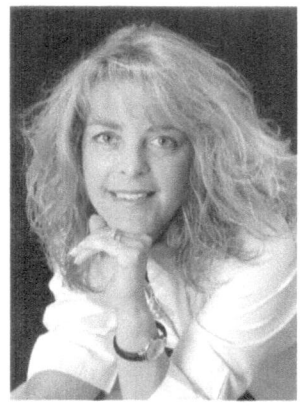

MICHELE TUCKER was born and raised in Virginia in the mid-60's. Her immediate family includes her husband of 16 years and teenage son, her mother, brother, one niece and one nephew.

Her 25-year career in the administrative field has taught her many personal lessons regarding how to act and react to pressure and crisis. Many supervisors she has had over the years have made a tremendous impact on her life for which she is eternally grateful.

In this her first novel, Michele writes of her passion to save her father from this terrible fate. Sadly, no matter how strong her passion, it was no match for the disease.

Michele is currently writing her second novel based on the tragic murder of her relative in Washington DC.

Michele would like to extend her sympathy and best wishes to those who are suffering this disease.